Healthy and Fit at 40: Eating Habits for a Strong Body and Mind

Introduction

Chapter 1: Introduction to Eating Habits for Health and Fitness at 40

Chapter 2: Plant-Based Eating Habits for Optimal Health in Your 40's

Chapter 3: Low-Carb Eating Habits for Weight Management in Your 40's

Chapter 4: Intermittent Fasting Eating Habits for Increased Energy in Your 40's

Chapter 5: Mediterranean Diet Eating Habits for Heart Health in Your 40's

Chapter 6: Gluten-Free Eating Habits for Digestive Health in Your 40's

Introduction

Entering your 40s often brings a renewed focus on health and wellness, as our bodies and lifestyles undergo significant changes. This book is designed to be your comprehensive guide to adopting and maintaining healthy eating habits that cater specifically to the unique needs of individuals in their 40s. Each chapter offers a detailed exploration of various dietary approaches, providing you with the knowledge and tools to optimize your health and fitness.

We begin by examining the importance of mindful eating habits and their impact on overall health and fitness. As you navigate through your 40s, establishing a solid foundation of healthy eating can enhance your quality of life, energy levels, and long-term well-being.

Plant-based eating habits are gaining popularity for their numerous health benefits. This book delves into how a plant-based diet can support optimal health, offering practical tips and delicious recipes to help you transition smoothly.

Weight management becomes increasingly important in your 40s, and low-carb eating habits can play a crucial role in achieving and maintaining a healthy weight. You'll discover effective strategies for incorporating low-carb meals into your daily routine without sacrificing flavour or satisfaction.

Intermittent fasting is another powerful tool for boosting energy levels and promoting overall health. This book provides insights into how intermittent fasting can be tailored to suit your lifestyle and enhance your vitality.

Heart health is a priority as we age, and the Mediterranean diet is renowned for its heart-healthy benefits. Learn how to incorporate this diet into your life to support cardiovascular health and enjoy a wide array of delicious foods.

Digestive health is crucial, and a gluten-free diet can alleviate many common digestive issues. Explore the benefits of going gluten-free and how to implement it effectively.

Maintaining muscle mass is vital, and protein-rich eating habits are essential for muscle maintenance. This book offers guidance on incorporating sufficient protein into your diet to support strength and vitality.

Reducing inflammation is key to preventing chronic diseases, and sugar-free eating habits can significantly contribute to this goal. Discover how to minimize sugar intake and enjoy a diet that supports inflammation reduction.

Stress management through mindful eating is another focus of this book. Learn techniques to cultivate mindful eating habits that help manage stress and promote mental well-being.

Balancing macro-nutrients is crucial for overall wellness. This book provides insights into achieving a balanced diet that supports all aspects of your health.

Finally, superfoods are celebrated for their immune-boosting properties. Learn how to incorporate these nutritional powerhouses into your diet to enhance your immune system.

Embark on this journey towards healthier eating habits and make lasting changes that will benefit you for years to come. This book is your essential companion for achieving and maintaining optimal health in your 40s.

Chapter 1: Introduction to Eating Habits for Health and Fitness at 40

As we reach our 40s, it is more important than ever to pay attention to our eating habits in order to maintain a strong body and mind. The choices we make when it comes to food can have a significant impact on our overall health and well-being. In this chapter, we will explore different eating habits that can help you stay healthy and fit in your 40s.

One of the key eating habits to consider in your 40s is adopting a plant-based diet. Plant-based eating has been shown to provide a wide range of health benefits, including reduced risk of chronic diseases such as heart disease, diabetes, and cancer. By incorporating more fruits, vegetables, whole grains, and legumes into your diet, you can improve your overall health and well-being.

Another important eating habit to consider in your 40s is following a low-carb diet for weight management. Cutting back on carbohydrates can help you maintain a healthy weight and reduce your risk of obesity-related health issues. By focusing on lean proteins, healthy fats, and non-starchy vegetables, you can support your weight loss goals and improve your overall health.

Intermittent fasting is another eating habit that can be beneficial for increasing energy levels in your 40s. By incorporating periods of fasting into your routine, you can improve your metabolism, boost your energy levels, and support your overall health. This eating habit can also help regulate blood sugar levels and reduce inflammation in the body.

In this chapter, we will also explore other eating habits such as following a Mediterranean diet for heart health, adopting a gluten-free diet for digestive health, and incorporating protein-rich foods for muscle maintenance. By making informed choices about your eating habits in your 40s, you can support your overall wellness and enjoy a strong body and mind for years to come.

Chapter 2: Plant-Based Eating Habits for Optimal Health in Your 40's

Benefits of a Plant-Based Diet

As we age, it becomes increasingly important to pay attention to our dietary choices in order to maintain optimal health and fitness. One dietary approach that has gained popularity in recent years is the plant-based diet. This eating pattern focuses on consuming predominantly plant-based foods such as fruits, vegetables, whole grains, nuts, seeds, and legumes, while minimizing or eliminating animal products. The benefits of a plant-based diet for individuals over 40 are numerous and can have a profound impact on overall health and well-being.

One of the primary benefits of a plant-based diet for individuals over 40 is its potential to reduce the risk of chronic diseases such as heart disease, diabetes, and certain types of cancer. Plant-based foods are rich in vitamins, minerals, antioxidants, and fibre, all of which play a crucial role in maintaining a healthy body and mind. By incorporating more plant-based foods into your diet, you can help lower cholesterol levels, regulate blood sugar, and reduce inflammation, all of which are key factors in preventing and managing chronic diseases.

In addition to reducing the risk of chronic diseases, a plant-based diet can also help individuals over 40 maintain a healthy weight. Plant-based foods are typically lower in calories and saturated fats than animal products, making them an excellent choice for those looking to manage their weight. By focusing on whole, unprocessed plant foods, you can feel satisfied and nourished while also supporting your weight management goals.

Furthermore, a plant-based diet can provide individuals over 40 with increased energy and vitality. Plant foods are rich in complex carbohydrates, which are the body's preferred source of fuel. By incorporating a variety of fruits, vegetables, whole grains, and legumes into your diet, you can help stabilize your blood sugar levels and maintain sustained energy throughout the day. This can be especially beneficial for those experiencing fatigue or low energy levels as they age.

Another benefit of a plant-based diet for individuals over 40 is its potential to support cognitive function and mental health. Research has shown that plant-based diets high in fruits, vegetables, and whole grains are associated with a reduced risk of cognitive decline and improved mood. By nourishing your brain with nutrient-dense plant foods, you can support cognitive function, memory, and overall mental well-being as you age.

In conclusion, a plant-based diet offers numerous benefits for individuals over 40 looking to maintain optimal health and fitness. By focusing on plant foods and minimizing animal products, you can reduce the risk of chronic diseases, manage your weight, increase energy levels, and support cognitive function. Consider incorporating more plant-based foods into your diet to reap the many benefits of this eating pattern for a strong body and mind in your 40s and beyond.

How to Incorporate More Plants into Your Diet

Incorporating more plants into your diet is a great way to boost your overall health and well-being, especially as you navigate through your 40s. Plant-based eating habits can provide you with a wide array of essential nutrients, fibre, and antioxidants that are beneficial for maintaining a strong body and mind. By focusing on incorporating more fruits, vegetables, whole grains, nuts, seeds, and legumes into your meals, you can support your body's natural processes and promote optimal health in your 40s.

One way to start incorporating more plants into your diet is by gradually increasing the amount of fruits and vegetables you consume each day. Aim to fill half of your plate with colourful fruits and vegetables at each meal to ensure you are getting a variety of vitamins, minerals, and antioxidants. You can also experiment with different cooking methods, such as roasting, steaming, or stir-frying, to enhance the flavors and textures of your plant-based dishes.

Another important aspect of incorporating more plants into your diet is to focus on whole grains, nuts, seeds, and legumes as sources of protein, fibre, and healthy fats. These plant-based foods can help you feel fuller for longer, stabilize your blood sugar levels, and support your digestive health. Try incorporating quinoa, brown rice, chia seeds, and lentils into your meals to add a plant-based protein boost and increase the nutrient density of your diet.

In addition to increasing your intake of plant-based foods, it is important to pay attention to the quality of your food choices. Opt for organic, locally sourced, and minimally processed plant-based foods whenever possible to ensure you are getting the most nutrients and benefits from your diet. By choosing whole, unprocessed foods, you can reduce your exposure to harmful chemicals, pesticides, and additives that can negatively impact your health in your 40s.

Overall, incorporating more plants into your diet can have a profound impact on your health and well-being in your 40s. By focusing on a variety of fruits, vegetables, whole grains, nuts, seeds, and legumes, you can support your body's natural processes, boost your energy levels, and promote optimal health. Remember to experiment with different plant-based foods, cooking methods, and meal combinations to find what works best for your body and lifestyle. By making small, sustainable changes to your diet, you can enjoy the benefits of a plant-based diet and maintain a strong body and mind well into your 40s and beyond.

Plant-Based Meal Planning Tips

Plant-based meal planning can be a great way to improve your overall health and well-being in your 40's. By focusing on incorporating more fruits, vegetables, whole grains, nuts, seeds, and legumes into your diet, you can ensure that you are getting a wide variety of essential nutrients that are beneficial for your body. When planning your meals, try to include a variety of colours on your plate to ensure that you are getting a diverse range of vitamins and minerals.

One important tip for plant-based meal planning is to make sure that you are getting an adequate amount of protein in your diet. While animal products are a common source of protein, there are plenty of plant-based sources as well, such as tofu, tempeh, lentils, beans, and quinoa. Including a variety of these protein-rich foods in your meals can help to ensure that you are meeting your daily protein needs.

Another tip for plant-based meal planning is to focus on whole foods rather than processed foods. Whole foods are generally more nutrient-dense and can help to keep you feeling full and satisfied throughout the day. Try to avoid overly processed plant-based foods, such as vegan junk food, and instead opt for whole grains, fruits, vegetables, and legumes.

When planning your plant-based meals, it can also be helpful to think about balance and variety. Try to include a mix of different food groups in each meal, such as carbohydrates, protein, healthy fats, and plenty of fruits and vegetables. By focusing on balance and variety, you can ensure that you are getting all of the essential nutrients that your body needs to thrive.

Overall, plant-based meal planning can be a great way to improve your health and well-being in your 40's. By focusing on whole, nutrient-dense foods, getting an adequate amount of protein, and ensuring balance and variety in your meals, you can set yourself up for success in maintaining a healthy and fit lifestyle. Experiment with different plant-based recipes and ingredients to keep things interesting and enjoyable, and remember that small changes can lead to big improvements in your overall health.

Chapter 3: Low-Carb Eating Habits for Weight Management in Your 40's

Understanding Carbohydrates and Weight Gain

Carbohydrates are a crucial component of our diet, providing our bodies with the energy needed to function properly. However, understanding the role of carbohydrates in weight gain is essential for maintaining a healthy and fit body in your 40s. Carbohydrates come in different forms, including simple sugars found in fruits and sweets, as well as complex carbohydrates found in whole grains, vegetables, and legumes. While carbohydrates are necessary for our bodies to function, consuming an excess amount can lead to weight gain.

When it comes to weight management in your 40s, it is important to be mindful of your carbohydrate intake. Opting for whole, unprocessed carbohydrates such as whole grains, fruits, and vegetables can help regulate blood sugar levels and prevent spikes that can lead to weight gain. On the other hand, consuming refined carbohydrates like white bread, sugary snacks, and processed foods can contribute to weight gain and other health issues.

One popular eating habit for weight management in your 40s is following a low-carb diet. By reducing your intake of carbohydrates and focusing on protein and healthy fats, you can effectively manage your weight and improve your overall health. Low-carb diets have been shown to be effective in promoting weight loss and reducing the risk of chronic diseases such as diabetes and heart disease.

Another eating habit that can aid in weight management and increase energy levels in your 40s is intermittent fasting. This eating pattern involves cycling between periods of eating and fasting, which can help regulate blood sugar levels, promote weight loss, and increase energy levels. By incorporating intermittent fasting into your routine, you can support your weight management goals and improve your overall health in your 40s.

In conclusion, understanding the relationship between carbohydrates and weight gain is essential for maintaining a healthy and fit body in your 40s. By being mindful of your carbohydrate intake, opting for whole, unprocessed carbohydrates, following a low-carb diet, and incorporating intermittent fasting into your eating habits, you can effectively manage your weight and improve your overall health. Remember to consult with a healthcare professional before making any significant changes to your diet to ensure that it aligns with your individual health needs and goals.

Low-Carb Food Options

When it comes to maintaining a healthy and fit body in your 40s, one important aspect to consider is your food choices. Low-carb food options can be a great way to manage weight and improve overall health. By reducing your intake of carbohydrates, you can help regulate blood sugar levels, reduce inflammation, and promote weight loss.

Some low-carb food options to consider include lean proteins such as chicken, turkey, and fish. These protein-rich foods can help maintain muscle mass and keep you feeling full and satisfied. Additionally, incorporating healthy fats like avocados, nuts, and seeds can provide essential nutrients and promote satiety.

Vegetables are another important component of a low-carb diet. Non-starchy vegetables such as leafy greens, broccoli, and cauliflower are high in fibre and vitamins, making them a nutritious and filling option. By including a variety of colourful vegetables in your meals, you can ensure you are getting a wide range of nutrients to support your overall health.

When planning your meals, consider incorporating low-carb swaps for high-carb foods. For example, instead of pasta, try using spiralized zucchini or spaghetti squash as a base for your favorite sauces. Cauliflower rice can also be a great substitute for traditional rice, offering a lower carb alternative that is just as satisfying.

Overall, choosing low-carb food options can help support weight management, improve energy levels, and promote overall wellness in your 40s. By focusing on nutrient-dense foods and making mindful choices, you can enjoy the benefits of a low-carb diet while maintaining a strong body and mind well into your 40s and beyond.

Tips for Success on a Low-Carb Diet

Following a low-carb diet can be a highly effective way to manage your weight, improve your overall health, and increase your energy levels in your 40s. However, sticking to a low-carb eating plan can be challenging at times. Here are some tips for success on a low-carb diet to help you stay on track and achieve your health and fitness goals.

First and foremost, it's important to focus on whole, nutrient-dense foods when following a low-carb diet. This means incorporating plenty of vegetables, lean proteins, healthy fats, and low-sugar fruits into your meals. By choosing these foods, you'll not only keep your carb intake in check but also provide your body with the essential nutrients it needs to thrive.

Another tip for success on a low-carb diet is to plan ahead and prepare your meals in advance. Having healthy, low-carb options readily available can help prevent you from reaching for high-carb, processed foods when you're hungry or short on time. Consider meal prepping on weekends or evenings to set yourself up for success throughout the week.

In addition, it's important to stay hydrated and drink plenty of water when following a low-carb diet. Drinking water can help curb cravings, support digestion, and keep you feeling full and satisfied between meals. Aim to drink at least eight glasses of water per day, and consider adding lemon or cucumber slices for a refreshing twist.

Furthermore, listen to your body and adjust your low-carb eating plan as needed. Everyone's nutritional needs are different, so pay attention to how your body responds to different foods and adjust your carb intake accordingly. If you find yourself feeling fatigued or sluggish on a low-carb diet, consider adding more healthy carbs like sweet potatoes or quinoa to your meals.

Lastly, don't be too hard on yourself if you slip up or indulge in a high-carb treat from time to time. Remember that balance is key, and it's important to enjoy your food and listen to your body's cravings in moderation. By following these tips for success on a low-carb diet, you can optimize your health and fitness in your 40s and beyond.

Chapter 4: Intermittent Fasting Eating Habits for Increased Energy in Your 40's

What is Intermittent Fasting?

Intermittent fasting is a popular eating pattern that involves cycling between periods of eating and fasting. This method has gained popularity in recent years for its potential health benefits, including weight loss, improved metabolic health, and increased energy levels. For those in their 40s, intermittent fasting can be a valuable tool for maintaining a strong body and mind.

There are several different methods of intermittent fasting, including the 16/8 method, where you fast for 16 hours and eat during an 8-hour window, and the 5:2 method, where you eat normally for 5 days a week and restrict calories on the other 2 days. These methods can be tailored to fit your lifestyle and preferences, making intermittent fasting a flexible and sustainable eating habit for those in their 40s.

One of the key benefits of intermittent fasting is its ability to promote weight loss and weight management. By limiting the window of time in which you eat, you may naturally consume fewer calories, leading to a reduction in body fat. Additionally, intermittent fasting has been shown to improve insulin sensitivity, which can help regulate blood sugar levels and reduce the risk of developing type 2 diabetes - a common concern for many in their 40s.

Intermittent fasting has also been linked to improvements in cognitive function and brain health. Fasting has been shown to increase the production of a protein called brain-derived neurotrophic factor (BDNF), which plays a key role in promoting the growth of new brain cells and protecting existing ones. This can help improve memory, focus, and overall cognitive function - important factors for maintaining a sharp mind in your 40s.

Overall, intermittent fasting can be a valuable addition to your eating habits in your 40s, offering a range of potential health benefits. Whether you're looking to manage your weight, boost your energy levels, or improve your cognitive function, intermittent fasting can be a powerful tool to help you achieve your health and fitness goals. Consider incorporating intermittent fasting into your routine and see how it can positively impact your body and mind in your 40s and beyond.

Benefits of Intermittent Fasting

Intermittent fasting has gained popularity in recent years as a way to improve health and increase energy levels. This eating habit involves cycling between periods of eating and fasting, with the goal of giving the digestive system a break and allowing the body to burn stored fat for energy. For individuals over 40, intermittent fasting can offer a range of benefits that contribute to overall health and well-being.

One of the key benefits of intermittent fasting for individuals over 40 is improved metabolic health. As we age, our metabolism naturally slows down, making it easier to gain weight and harder to lose it. Intermittent fasting can help to kick-start the metabolism and promote weight loss by increasing the body's ability to burn fat for fuel. This can lead to a reduction in body fat, particularly around the abdominal area, which is important for reducing the risk of chronic diseases such as diabetes and heart disease.

Intermittent fasting has also been shown to have positive effects on brain health and cognitive function. Fasting has been found to increase the production of brain-derived neurotrophic factor (BDNF), a protein that promotes the growth and survival of nerve cells. This can help to improve memory, focus, and overall brain function, which is especially important for individuals over 40 who may be experiencing age-related cognitive decline. In addition, intermittent fasting has been linked to a reduced risk of neurodegenerative diseases such as Alzheimer's and Parkinson's.

Another benefit of intermittent fasting for individuals over 40 is improved insulin sensitivity. Insulin is a hormone that regulates blood sugar levels, and insulin resistance is a common issue as we age. By giving the body regular breaks from eating, intermittent fasting can help to lower blood sugar levels and improve insulin sensitivity, which is important for reducing the risk of type 2 diabetes and other metabolic disorders. This can also lead to a reduction in inflammation in the body, which is a key factor in many chronic diseases.

In addition to the physical benefits, intermittent fasting can also have positive effects on mental health and emotional well-being. Fasting has been found to reduce stress levels and improve mood by increasing the production of feel-good hormones such as serotonin and dopamine. This can help individuals over 40 to better manage stress, anxiety, and depression, which are common issues in this age group. By promoting a sense of calm and balance, intermittent fasting can contribute to overall mental wellness and emotional resilience.

Overall, intermittent fasting is a powerful eating habit that can offer a range of benefits for individuals over 40. From improved metabolic health and weight management to enhanced brain function and emotional well-being, intermittent fasting has the potential to transform your health and vitality. By incorporating this eating habit into your daily routine, you can take control of your health and well-being in your 40s and beyond.

How to Start Intermittent Fasting Safely

Intermittent fasting is a popular eating pattern that involves cycling between periods of eating and fasting. It has been shown to have numerous health benefits, including weight loss, improved metabolic health, and increased energy levels. However, it is important to approach intermittent fasting with caution, especially if you are over 40 years old. Here are some tips on how to start intermittent fasting safely.

First and foremost, it is important to consult with a healthcare professional before starting any new eating regimen, especially if you have any underlying health conditions or are taking medications. They can help you determine if intermittent fasting is right for you and provide guidance on how to safely incorporate it into your lifestyle.

When starting intermittent fasting, it is important to start slowly and gradually increase the fasting periods over time. This will allow your body to adjust to the new eating pattern and minimize any negative side effects, such as fatigue or irritability. Start by fasting for 12 hours overnight and gradually increase the fasting window to 14-16 hours over a period of weeks.

During the fasting periods, it is important to stay hydrated and consume plenty of water to help curb hunger and support your body's natural detoxification processes. You can also consume calorie-free beverages such as herbal tea or black coffee to help suppress appetite.

It is also important to focus on nutrient-dense foods during your eating periods to ensure that you are getting all the essential vitamins and minerals your body needs. Incorporate plenty of fruits, vegetables, whole grains, lean proteins, and healthy fats into your meals to support overall health and well-being.

Lastly, listen to your body and adjust your fasting schedule as needed. If you experience any negative side effects or if intermittent fasting does not feel right for you, it is okay to stop or modify your approach. Remember, the goal is to find an eating pattern that works for you and supports your health and fitness goals in your 40s and beyond.

Chapter 5: Mediterranean Diet Eating Habits for Heart Health in Your 40's

Key Components of the Mediterranean Diet

The Mediterranean diet is a popular eating plan that has been associated with numerous health benefits, particularly for individuals over the age of 40. This diet is based on the traditional eating habits of people living in countries bordering the Mediterranean Sea, such as Greece, Italy, and Spain. The key components of the Mediterranean diet include an emphasis on whole, minimally processed foods, such as fruits, vegetables, whole grains, nuts, seeds, and legumes.

One of the main principles of the Mediterranean diet is the consumption of healthy fats, such as olive oil, nuts, and fatty fish. These fats are rich in monounsaturated and omega-3 fatty acids, which have been shown to have numerous health benefits, including reducing inflammation, improving heart health, and supporting brain function. Additionally, the Mediterranean diet is rich in antioxidants, which help protect the body from oxidative stress and reduce the risk of chronic diseases such as cancer and heart disease.

Another key component of the Mediterranean diet is the inclusion of lean protein sources, such as poultry, fish, and legumes. Protein is essential for muscle maintenance and repair, especially as we age. By including lean protein in your diet, you can support muscle strength and function, which is important for overall health and mobility in your 40s and beyond. Additionally, the Mediterranean diet emphasizes the importance of eating a variety of colourful fruits and vegetables, which are rich in vitamins, minerals, and phytonutrients that support optimal health and well-being.

In addition to the specific foods included in the Mediterranean diet, another important component is the emphasis on meal timing and portion control. The Mediterranean diet encourages regular, balanced meals and snacks throughout the day, with an emphasis on listening to your body's hunger and fullness cues. This approach can help prevent overeating and promote better digestion and nutrient absorption. Furthermore, the Mediterranean diet is not just about what you eat, but also how you eat. The diet emphasizes the importance of enjoying meals with family and friends, savouring each bite, and being mindful of your eating habits, which can help reduce stress and improve overall well-being in your 40s.

Overall, the Mediterranean diet is a well-rounded eating plan that can help individuals over the age of 40 maintain a strong body and mind. By incorporating key components of the Mediterranean diet, such as whole, minimally processed foods, healthy fats, lean proteins, and colourful fruits and vegetables, you can support heart health, reduce inflammation, maintain muscle mass, and improve overall well-being. Additionally, the Mediterranean diet promotes mindful eating habits, which can help reduce stress and support mental health in your 40s and beyond. Consider incorporating elements of the Mediterranean diet into your eating habits to keep you healthy and fit as you age.

Health Benefits of the Mediterranean Diet

The Mediterranean diet is often hailed as one of the healthiest eating habits for individuals over 40. This diet is based on the traditional foods and cooking styles of countries bordering the Mediterranean Sea, such as Greece, Italy, and Spain. It emphasizes the consumption of fruits, vegetables, whole grains, legumes, nuts, and healthy fats like olive oil. By following the Mediterranean diet, individuals can experience a wide range of health benefits that can help them maintain a strong body and mind well into their 40s and beyond.

One of the key health benefits of the Mediterranean diet is its ability to promote heart health. The diet is rich in foods that are known to reduce the risk of heart disease, such as olive oil, nuts, and fatty fish. These foods are high in monounsaturated fats and omega-3 fatty acids, which can help lower cholesterol levels and reduce inflammation in the body. By incorporating these heart-healthy foods into their meals, individuals can support their cardiovascular health and reduce their risk of heart-related issues as they age.

In addition to promoting heart health, the Mediterranean diet is also beneficial for weight management in individuals over 40. The diet is focused on whole, nutrient-dense foods that are low in processed sugars and unhealthy fats. By following this eating pattern, individuals can naturally control their calorie intake and maintain a healthy weight. The diet is also high in fibre, which can help individuals feel fuller for longer periods of time and prevent overeating. By adopting the Mediterranean diet, individuals can support their weight management goals and maintain a healthy body composition well into their 40s.

Furthermore, the Mediterranean diet is known for its anti-inflammatory properties, which can help reduce inflammation in the body and support overall wellness. Many of the foods included in this diet, such as fruits, vegetables, and olive oil, are rich in antioxidants and polyphenols that can help combat inflammation and oxidative stress. By incorporating these foods into their meals, individuals can support their immune system, reduce their risk of chronic diseases, and promote overall well-being. The Mediterranean diet's focus on whole, minimally processed foods can also help individuals reduce their intake of inflammatory foods, such as refined sugars and trans fats, which can contribute to inflammation in the body.

Overall, the Mediterranean diet is a well-rounded eating pattern that can benefit individuals over 40 in numerous ways. From promoting heart health and weight management to reducing inflammation and supporting overall wellness, this diet offers a wide range of health benefits that can help individuals maintain a strong body and mind as they age. By incorporating the principles of the Mediterranean diet into their daily eating habits, individuals can improve their health, increase their energy levels, and enjoy a higher quality of life well into their 40s and beyond.

Mediterranean Diet Meal Ideas

The Mediterranean diet is renowned for its health benefits, particularly in promoting heart health and overall well-being. Incorporating Mediterranean diet meal ideas into your daily routine can help you maintain a strong body and mind in your 40s. This diet emphasizes whole, unprocessed foods such as fruits, vegetables, whole grains, legumes, nuts, seeds, and olive oil. It also includes moderate amounts of fish and poultry, with red meat consumed sparingly.

One delicious Mediterranean diet meal idea is a Greek salad with grilled chicken. This refreshing dish features a mix of fresh vegetables like cucumbers, tomatoes, and bell peppers, topped with feta cheese and olives. The grilled chicken adds a protein boost and makes this salad a satisfying meal. Drizzle with olive oil and a squeeze of lemon for a flavourful dressing.

Another Mediterranean-inspired meal idea is a quinoa and chickpea Buddha bowl. This plant-based dish is packed with protein and fibre, thanks to the quinoa and chickpeas. Add in a variety of colourful vegetables such as roasted sweet potatoes, cherry tomatoes, and spinach. Top with a dollop of hummus and a sprinkle of fresh herbs for a nourishing and satisfying meal.

For a low-carb Mediterranean meal idea, try grilled shrimp with zucchini noodles. This light and flavourful dish features succulent shrimp marinated in lemon, garlic, and herbs, served over spiralized zucchini noodles. The combination of seafood and vegetables provides a nutrient-rich meal that is low in carbohydrates but high in essential vitamins and minerals.

Intermittent fasting is a popular eating habit for increased energy in your 40s. You can incorporate the principles of the Mediterranean diet into your fasting routine by enjoying a hearty breakfast of Greek yogurt with berries and nuts. This protein-rich meal will keep you feeling full and energized throughout the morning, making it easier to stick to your fasting schedule. By combining the benefits of intermittent fasting with the nutrient-dense foods of the Mediterranean diet, you can support your body's natural energy production and overall vitality.

Chapter 6: Gluten-Free Eating Habits for Digestive Health in Your 40's

Understanding Gluten Sensitivity and Celiac Disease

Gluten sensitivity and celiac disease are two conditions that involve adverse reactions to gluten, a protein found in wheat, barley, and rye. While both conditions share some similarities, they differ in their severity and underlying mechanisms. Gluten sensitivity, also known as non-celiac gluten sensitivity, is a less severe condition that can cause symptoms such as bloating, fatigue, and headaches. On the other hand, celiac disease is an autoimmune disorder in which the ingestion of gluten leads to damage in the small intestine.

Individuals over the age of 40 may be more susceptible to developing gluten sensitivity or celiac disease due to changes in their digestive system and immune response. It is important for this age group to be aware of the symptoms of these conditions and to seek proper diagnosis and treatment if necessary. Symptoms of gluten sensitivity and celiac disease can vary widely and may include digestive issues, skin rashes, joint pain, and neurological symptoms.

For individuals in their 40s who suspect they may have gluten sensitivity or celiac disease, it is recommended to consult with a healthcare provider for proper testing and diagnosis. Testing for celiac disease typically involves blood tests to check for specific antibodies, as well as an endoscopy to examine the small intestine for damage. In the case of gluten sensitivity, diagnosis may be more challenging, as there are currently no specific tests available. However, individuals can try an elimination diet to see if symptoms improve when gluten is removed from their diet.

In conclusion, understanding gluten sensitivity and celiac disease is crucial for individuals over 40 who are looking to maintain a healthy and fit lifestyle. By being aware of the symptoms and seeking proper diagnosis and treatment, individuals can effectively manage these conditions and improve their overall well-being. It is important to consult with a healthcare provider for personalized guidance and support in navigating gluten-related issues.

Gluten-Free Food Swaps

For those in their 40s looking to maintain a healthy and fit lifestyle, making small changes to your diet can have a big impact. One popular dietary trend that has gained traction in recent years is gluten-free eating. Gluten is a protein found in wheat, barley, and rye that can cause digestive issues for some individuals. By making gluten-free food swaps, you can improve your digestive health and overall well-being.

When it comes to gluten-free food swaps, there are plenty of delicious and nutritious options available. Instead of traditional wheat pasta, opt for gluten-free alternatives like brown rice pasta or chickpea pasta. These options are just as satisfying and can help prevent bloating and discomfort. Similarly, swap out wheat flour for almond flour or coconut flour in your baking recipes to create gluten-free treats that are just as tasty.

In addition to pasta and baking, there are plenty of other gluten-free food swaps you can make in your daily meals.

Instead of sandwiches on wheat bread, try using lettuce wraps or gluten-free bread made from ingredients like quinoa or flaxseed. For breakfast, swap out traditional cereal for gluten-free options like oatmeal, quinoa, or chia seed pudding. These swaps can help you maintain a balanced and nutritious diet while avoiding gluten.

It's important to note that not all gluten-free products are created equal. Some gluten-free packaged foods can be high in sugar, unhealthy fats, and preservatives. As you make gluten-free food swaps, be sure to read labels carefully and choose whole, unprocessed foods whenever possible. By opting for naturally gluten-free foods like fruits, vegetables, lean proteins, and whole grains, you can ensure that you are maintaining a healthy and balanced diet.

Overall, making gluten-free food swaps can be a beneficial choice for those in their 40s looking to improve their digestive health and overall well-being. By choosing nutrient-dense, whole foods and avoiding processed gluten-free products, you can support your body's needs and feel your best. Experiment with different gluten-free swaps in your meals and snacks to find what works best for you and enjoy the benefits of a gluten-free lifestyle in your 40s.

Gluten-Free Recipes

When it comes to maintaining good digestive health in your 40s, gluten-free eating habits can play a significant role. For individuals with gluten sensitivities or celiac disease, avoiding gluten is crucial to prevent gastrointestinal discomfort and other health issues. Fortunately, there are plenty of delicious and nutritious gluten-free recipes that can help you stay healthy and fit at this stage of life.

One popular gluten-free recipe to try is quinoa salad with roasted vegetables. Quinoa is a versatile grain that is naturally gluten-free and packed with protein and essential nutrients. By combining it with a variety of colourful roasted vegetables such as bell peppers, zucchini, and cherry tomatoes, you can create a tasty and satisfying meal that is perfect for lunch or dinner. Drizzle with a homemade vinaigrette made with olive oil, lemon juice, and herbs for added flavour.

Another gluten-free recipe option is cauliflower crust pizza. Instead of traditional wheat-based pizza crust, this recipe uses cauliflower as the base, making it a great low-carb alternative. Simply pulse cauliflower in a food processor, then mix with eggs, cheese, and seasonings to form a dough. Top with your favorite pizza toppings such as tomato sauce, cheese, and vegetables, then bake until golden and crispy. This guilt-free pizza is a delicious way to satisfy your cravings without compromising your gluten-free diet.

For a sweet treat that won't derail your gluten-free eating habits, try making almond flour banana bread. Almond flour is a nutritious gluten-free alternative to traditional wheat flour, and when combined with ripe bananas, eggs, and a touch of honey, it creates a moist and flavourful bread that is perfect for breakfast or snacking. Feel free to add in extras such as chopped nuts, dried fruit, or chocolate chips for added texture and flavour.

In conclusion, incorporating gluten-free recipes into your eating habits can help support your digestive health and overall well-being in your 40s. Whether you're looking for savoury meals like quinoa salad with roasted vegetables, indulgent treats like cauliflower crust pizza, or wholesome snacks like almond flour banana bread, there are plenty of delicious options to choose from. Experiment with different ingredients and flavors to find gluten-free recipes that you enjoy and that nourish your body and mind.

Chapter 7: Protein-Rich Eating Habits for Muscle Maintenance in Your 40's

Importance of Protein for Muscle Health

Protein is an essential nutrient for maintaining muscle health, especially as we age. As individuals over 40, it is important to prioritize protein-rich foods in our diets to support muscle maintenance and overall physical well-being. Protein plays a crucial role in repairing and building muscle tissue, making it essential for those looking to stay healthy and fit in their 40s.

Adequate protein intake is particularly important for individuals engaging in physical activity or strength training, as it helps to promote muscle growth and repair. As we age, our bodies may become less efficient at utilizing protein, making it even more crucial to ensure we are consuming enough of this nutrient to support muscle health. Including protein-rich foods such as lean meats, poultry, fish, eggs, dairy products, legumes, nuts, and seeds in our diets can help us meet our protein needs and maintain strong, healthy muscles.

In addition to supporting muscle health, protein also plays a role in weight management and satiety. High-protein foods are known to help keep us feeling full and satisfied, which can aid in weight loss or maintenance efforts. By including protein-rich foods in our meals and snacks, we can help prevent overeating and support our overall health and fitness goals in our 40s.

For those following plant-based eating habits, there are plenty of protein-rich options available, such as tofu, tempeh, edamame, lentils, chickpeas, quinoa, and nuts. Incorporating a variety of plant-based protein sources into meals can help ensure that individuals following a vegetarian or vegan diet are meeting their protein needs and supporting muscle health in their 40s.

In conclusion, prioritizing protein-rich eating habits is essential for maintaining muscle health, supporting weight management, and promoting overall physical well-being in your 40s. By including a variety of protein sources in your diet and paying attention to your body's needs, you can help ensure that you are getting the nutrients necessary to stay healthy and fit as you age.

Protein-Rich Foods to Include in Your Diet

Protein is an essential nutrient that plays a crucial role in maintaining muscle mass, supporting immune function, and promoting overall health. As we age, it becomes even more important to ensure that we are consuming an adequate amount of protein in our diets. Including protein-rich foods in your meals can help you stay strong and healthy well into your 40s and beyond.

One of the best sources of protein is lean meats such as chicken, turkey, and fish. These foods are not only high in protein but also contain important nutrients like iron and omega-3 fatty acids. Including these lean meats in your diet can help you maintain muscle mass and support your body's repair and recovery processes.

Plant-based protein sources are also a great option for those looking to increase their protein intake. Foods like beans, lentils, tofu, and quinoa are all excellent sources of protein that can easily be incorporated into meals. Plant-based proteins are also rich in fibre, vitamins, and minerals, making them a nutritious choice for overall health and wellness.

For those looking to manage their weight in their 40s, incorporating low-carb protein-rich foods into their diet can be beneficial. Foods like eggs, Greek yogurt, and cottage cheese are low in carbohydrates but high in protein, making them a great choice for those looking to maintain a healthy weight. These foods can help you feel full and satisfied while also supporting muscle maintenance and repair.

Incorporating protein-rich foods into your diet can help you stay strong, healthy, and fit in your 40s. Whether you choose lean meats, plant-based proteins, or low-carb options, making protein a priority in your meals can have a positive impact on your overall health and well-being. By including a variety of protein-rich foods in your diet, you can ensure that you are getting the nutrients you need to thrive in your 40s and beyond.

Protein-Packed Meal Ideas

In your 40s, it is essential to focus on maintaining a strong and healthy body through proper nutrition. One important aspect of your diet should be ensuring that you are getting an adequate amount of protein in your meals. Protein is crucial for muscle maintenance, tissue repair, and overall health. Here are some protein-packed meal ideas to help you stay healthy and fit in your 40s.

One great option for a protein-packed meal is a quinoa salad with grilled chicken. Quinoa is a complete protein, meaning it contains all nine essential amino acids that our bodies need. Adding grilled chicken to the salad increases the protein content even further, making it a satisfying and nutritious meal. You can also add various vegetables and a light vinaigrette dressing to enhance the flavour and nutrient profile of the dish.

Another protein-rich meal idea is a tofu stir-fry with vegetables. Tofu is an excellent plant-based source of protein and is versatile enough to be used in a variety of dishes. Stir-frying tofu with colourful vegetables like bell peppers, broccoli, and snow peas not only adds a pop of flavour but also boosts the protein content of the meal. You can season the stir-fry with soy sauce, ginger, and garlic for a delicious and nutritious dish.

For a low-carb protein-packed meal, consider making a tuna and avocado salad. Tuna is a lean protein source that is also rich in omega-3 fatty acids, which are beneficial for heart health. Pairing it with creamy avocado adds even more protein and healthy fats to the dish. You can mix the tuna and avocado with leafy greens, cherry tomatoes, and a squeeze of lemon juice for a refreshing and nutrient-dense meal.

If you are looking to incorporate intermittent fasting into your eating habits for increased energy, a protein-rich smoothie can be a great option for a quick and convenient meal. Blend together protein powder, almond milk, frozen berries, spinach, and a tablespoon of nut butter for a delicious and filling smoothie that will keep you energized throughout the day. This meal is not only high in protein but also provides essential vitamins and minerals for optimal health.

Incorporating protein-rich foods into your diet is essential for muscle maintenance and overall wellness in your 40s. By including these protein-packed meal ideas in your eating habits, you can ensure that you are getting the nutrients your body needs to stay healthy and fit as you age. Experiment with different ingredients and recipes to find what works best for you and enjoy the benefits of a protein-rich diet for your body and mind.

Chapter 8: Sugar-Free Eating Habits for Reducing Inflammation in Your 40's

The Negative Effects of Sugar on Inflammation

Sugar is a common ingredient in many of the foods we consume on a daily basis, but its effects on inflammation can be detrimental to our health, especially as we age. Inflammation is the body's natural response to injury or infection, but chronic inflammation can lead to a host of health problems, including heart disease, diabetes, and arthritis. Consuming too much sugar can trigger inflammation in the body, leading to a cascade of negative effects on our overall health.

When we consume sugar, our bodies release inflammatory molecules called cytokines. These cytokines can increase the production of free radicals, which can damage cells and tissues in the body. This can lead to a state of chronic inflammation, which has been linked to a number of chronic diseases. By reducing our sugar intake, we can help decrease the levels of inflammation in our bodies and reduce our risk of developing these diseases.

One of the ways in which sugar contributes to inflammation is through its effect on insulin levels. When we consume sugar, our bodies release insulin to help regulate our blood sugar levels. However, consuming too much sugar can lead to insulin resistance, where our cells become less responsive to insulin. This can lead to higher levels of inflammation in the body, as well as an increased risk of developing type 2 diabetes.

In addition to its effects on insulin levels, sugar can also contribute to inflammation through its impact on the gut microbiome. The bacteria in our gut play a crucial role in regulating inflammation in the body, and consuming too much sugar can disrupt the balance of these bacteria. This can lead to an overgrowth of harmful bacteria, which can trigger inflammation in the gut and throughout the body. By reducing our sugar intake and consuming more fibre-rich foods, we can help support a healthy gut microbiome and reduce inflammation in the body.

Overall, reducing our sugar intake is an important step in reducing inflammation and improving our overall health, especially as we age. By making small changes to our diet, such as cutting back on sugary snacks and drinks, we can help reduce our risk of developing chronic diseases and improve our overall well-being. It's never too late to make healthier choices when it comes to our diet, and taking steps to reduce our sugar intake can have a lasting impact on our health and vitality in our 40s and beyond.

How to Reduce Sugar Intake

Reducing sugar intake is crucial for maintaining a healthy and fit body in your 40s. Excessive sugar consumption has been linked to a variety of health issues, including weight gain, inflammation, and an increased risk of chronic diseases such as diabetes and heart disease. By making small changes to your diet and lifestyle, you can significantly reduce your sugar intake and improve your overall well-being.

One of the easiest ways to reduce sugar intake is to cut back on sugary beverages such as soda, fruit juice, and energy drinks. These beverages are often loaded with added sugars and offer little to no nutritional value. Instead, opt for water, herbal teas, or unsweetened beverages to quench your thirst and stay hydrated throughout the day.

Another effective way to reduce sugar intake is to read food labels carefully and avoid products that contain high amounts of added sugars. Ingredients such as sucrose, high fructose corn syrup, and dextrose are all forms of added sugars that can contribute to excess sugar consumption. Choose whole foods such as fruits, vegetables, whole grains, and lean proteins that are naturally low in sugar and rich in essential nutrients.

Incorporating more whole foods into your diet can help you reduce your sugar intake while providing your body with the nutrients it needs to thrive. Fruits and vegetables are excellent sources of vitamins, minerals, and antioxidants that can support your overall health and well-being. Try to fill your plate with a variety of colourful fruits and vegetables to ensure you are getting a wide range of nutrients without the added sugars found in processed foods.

Lastly, be mindful of your sugar cravings and find healthier alternatives to satisfy your sweet tooth. Opt for naturally sweet foods such as berries, dates, or dark chocolate in moderation to curb your cravings without consuming excessive amounts of added sugars. By making conscious choices and being aware of your sugar intake, you can take control of your health and maintain a strong body and mind well into your 40s and beyond.

Sugar-Free Snack Ideas

When it comes to maintaining a healthy and fit lifestyle in your 40's, it's important to be mindful of your sugar intake. Excess sugar consumption has been linked to various health issues, including inflammation, weight gain, and increased risk of chronic diseases. In this subchapter, we will explore some delicious and satisfying sugar-free snack ideas that will keep you energized and feeling your best.

One great sugar-free snack option is a bowl of mixed nuts and seeds. Nuts and seeds are packed with healthy fats, protein, and fibre, making them a nutritious and filling choice. Try mixing almonds, walnuts, pumpkin seeds, and sunflower seeds for a tasty and satisfying snack. You can also add a sprinkle of cinnamon or a dash of sea salt for extra flavour.

Another delicious sugar-free snack idea is Greek yogurt with fresh berries. Greek yogurt is high in protein and probiotics, which are beneficial for gut health. Choose plain, unsweetened Greek yogurt and top it with a handful of fresh berries, such as blueberries, strawberries, or raspberries. Berries are low in sugar and high in antioxidants, making them a perfect addition to your snack.

For a savoury option, consider making cucumber and hummus bites. Cucumbers are low in calories and high in water content, making them a hydrating and refreshing snack. Pair cucumber slices with a dollop of hummus for a satisfying and nutritious treat. Hummus is made from chickpeas, which are a good source of protein and fibre, making it a great option for keeping you full and satisfied.

If you're craving something sweet, try a sugar-free chia pudding. Chia seeds are high in fibre and omega-3 fatty acids, making them a great addition to your diet. To make chia pudding, simply mix chia seeds with unsweetened almond milk and a dash of vanilla extract. Let it sit in the fridge overnight to thicken, then top it with fresh fruit or a sprinkle of unsweetened coconut flakes for a delicious and guilt-free snack.

Incorporating these sugar-free snack ideas into your daily routine can help you maintain a healthy and fit lifestyle in your 40's. By choosing nutrient-dense foods that are low in sugar, you can support your overall health and well-being. Experiment with different flavors and ingredients to find snacks that you enjoy and that leave you feeling satisfied and energized. Remember, small changes in your eating habits can have a big impact on your health in the long run.

Chapter 9: Mindful Eating Habits for Stress Management in Your 40's

Benefits of Mindful Eating

Mindful eating is a practice that involves paying full attention to the experience of eating and drinking, both inside and outside the body. This means being aware of the colours, smells, flavors, and textures of your food, as well as your body's hunger and fullness cues. By practicing mindful eating, you can develop a greater appreciation for the food you consume and make more conscious choices about what you eat.

One of the key benefits of mindful eating is that it can help you manage stress more effectively. When you take the time to savour each bite of your meal and focus on the present moment, you can reduce feelings of anxiety and overwhelm. By being fully present during the eating process, you can also prevent mindless eating, which often leads to overeating and negative emotions.

In addition to stress management, mindful eating can also support weight management in your 40's. By paying attention to your body's hunger and fullness signals, you can avoid mindless snacking and unnecessary calorie consumption. This can help you maintain a healthy weight and prevent weight gain as you age. Furthermore, mindful eating can help you develop a healthier relationship with food, leading to more balanced and sustainable eating habits.

Another benefit of mindful eating is improved digestion. When you take the time to chew your food thoroughly and appreciate each bite, you can promote better digestion and nutrient absorption. This can help prevent digestive issues such as bloating, gas, and indigestion. By being mindful of what you eat and how you eat it, you can support optimal digestive health and overall wellness in your 40's.

Overall, practicing mindful eating can enhance your overall well-being in your 40's. By being more present and intentional with your food choices, you can improve your relationship with food, manage stress more effectively, support weight management, and promote better digestion. Incorporating mindful eating habits into your daily routine can help you feel more connected to your body and make healthier choices that support your physical and mental health as you age.

Tips for Eating Mindfully

Eating mindfully is a practice that can greatly benefit your overall health and well-being, especially as you navigate through your 40s. Mindful eating involves paying attention to what you eat, how you eat, and why you eat. By being more aware of your eating habits, you can make better choices that support your body and mind. Here are some tips for incorporating mindful eating into your daily routine:

First and foremost, slow down and savour your meals. Take the time to chew your food thoroughly and really taste each bite. This not only helps with digestion but also allows you to fully experience the flavors and textures of your food. Eating slowly also gives your brain time to register when you are full, preventing overeating.

Another tip for eating mindfully is to eliminate distractions during meal times. Turn off the TV, put away your phone, and focus on the food in front of you. This allows you to be present in the moment and fully appreciate your meal. By being more mindful of your eating experience, you can better tune in to your body's hunger and fullness cues.

It's also important to listen to your body and eat when you are truly hungry. Avoid eating out of boredom or emotional reasons. Pay attention to physical hunger cues such as a growling stomach or low energy levels. By eating only when you are hungry, you can better regulate your food intake and maintain a healthy weight.

Incorporating a variety of colourful, whole foods into your diet is another key aspect of mindful eating. Fruits, vegetables, whole grains, lean proteins, and healthy fats provide essential nutrients that support your body's functions. Aim to fill your plate with a rainbow of fruits and vegetables to ensure you are getting a wide range of vitamins and minerals.

Lastly, practice gratitude for the food you are eating. Take a moment before each meal to express gratitude for the nourishment it provides your body. This simple practice can help you develop a deeper appreciation for the food you eat and cultivate a positive relationship with eating. By eating mindfully and with intention, you can support your health and well-being in your 40s and beyond.

Mindful Eating Practices for Stress Relief

Mindful eating practices can be a powerful tool for managing stress and promoting overall wellness, especially as we navigate the challenges of aging in our 40s. By paying attention to what and how we eat, we can cultivate a deeper connection with our bodies and minds, leading to reduced stress levels and improved mental clarity. Here are some key strategies for incorporating mindful eating into your daily routine to help you feel healthier and more balanced in your 40s.

One of the first steps in practicing mindful eating is to slow down and savour each bite. Take the time to appreciate the flavors, textures, and aromas of your food, rather than rushing through meals mindlessly. By eating slowly and mindfully, you can better tune into your body's hunger and fullness cues, which can help prevent overeating and promote healthier digestion. This practice can also help you feel more satisfied with smaller portions, leading to better weight management and improved overall health.

Another important aspect of mindful eating is being present and focused during meals. Avoid distractions like watching TV or scrolling through your phone while eating, as this can lead to mindless overeating and poor digestion. Instead, try to create a peaceful and calm environment for your meals, free from distractions and stress. By focusing on the act of eating and enjoying your food, you can cultivate a sense of gratitude and mindfulness that can help reduce stress and promote relaxation.

In addition to slowing down and being present during meals, it's also important to listen to your body's hunger and fullness signals. Pay attention to how your body feels before, during, and after eating, and adjust your portions accordingly. Eating when you're truly hungry and stopping when you're comfortably full can help you maintain a healthy weight and prevent emotional eating. By tuning into your body's natural cues, you can develop a more intuitive and mindful approach to eating that supports both physical and mental well-being.

Finally, practicing mindful eating can also involve being more aware of the emotional and psychological aspects of your relationship with food. Notice any patterns of emotional eating, stress-related cravings, or mindless snacking, and try to address these behaviours with compassion and self-awareness. By cultivating a more mindful and intentional approach to eating, you can develop a healthier and more balanced relationship with food that supports your overall wellness in your 40s and beyond.

Chapter 10: Balanced Macro-Nutrient Eating Habits for Overall Wellness in Your 40's

Understanding Macros: Proteins, Fats, and Carbs

Understanding macros - proteins, fats, and carbs - is essential for maintaining a healthy and fit body in your 40s. These three macronutrients play a crucial role in providing energy, supporting bodily functions, and maintaining overall health. By understanding how to balance these macros in your diet, you can optimize you're eating habits to support your body and mind as you age.

Proteins are the building blocks of life and are essential for muscle maintenance, repair, and growth. In your 40s, it is important to include protein-rich foods such as lean meats, poultry, fish, eggs, legumes, and dairy products in your diet. Aim to include a source of protein in every meal to support muscle health and keep you feeling full and satisfied throughout the day.

Fats are another important macronutrient that plays a vital role in hormone production, brain function, and nutrient absorption. In your 40s, focus on including healthy fats such as avocados, nuts, seeds, olive oil, and fatty fish in your diet. Avoiding trans fats and excessive saturated fats can help reduce inflammation and support heart health as you age.

Carbohydrates are the body's primary source of energy, but not all carbs are created equal. In your 40s, opt for complex carbohydrates such as whole grains, fruits, vegetables, and legumes to provide sustained energy and support digestive health. Limiting refined sugars and processed foods can help stabilize blood sugar levels and prevent energy crashes throughout the day.

By understanding the role of proteins, fats, and carbs in your diet, you can make informed choices to support your health and fitness goals in your 40s. Remember to focus on a balanced intake of all three macronutrients, along with plenty of fruits, vegetables, and whole foods, to promote overall wellness and longevity. Experiment with different eating habits, such as plant-based, low-carb, or intermittent fasting, to find what works best for your body and lifestyle in your 40s.

How to Achieve a Balanced Diet

Achieving a balanced diet is essential for maintaining good health and overall wellness, especially as we age. In our 40s, it becomes even more crucial to pay attention to what we eat in order to support our bodies and minds. By incorporating a variety of nutrient-dense foods into our daily meals, we can ensure that we are getting the essential vitamins and minerals needed for optimal health.

One way to achieve a balanced diet is by focusing on plant-based eating habits. This means incorporating plenty of fruits, vegetables, whole grains, nuts, and seeds into our meals. Plant-based foods are rich in antioxidants, fibre, and phytonutrients that can help reduce inflammation, boost immunity, and support overall health. By filling our plates with a colourful array of plant foods, we can ensure that we are getting a wide range of nutrients to support our bodies in our 40s.

In addition to plant-based eating, it is also important to consider low-carb eating habits for weight management in our 40s. By reducing our intake of refined carbohydrates and sugars, we can help stabilize blood sugar levels, promote weight loss, and improve overall energy levels. Opting for complex carbohydrates like whole grains, legumes, and vegetables can help keep us feeling full and satisfied while supporting our weight management goals.

Intermittent fasting is another eating habit that can be beneficial for increasing energy levels in our 40s. By incorporating periods of fasting into our daily routine, we can give our digestive system a break, improve insulin sensitivity, and promote fat burning. This can lead to increased energy levels, improved mental clarity, and better overall health.

Overall, achieving a balanced diet in our 40s requires a combination of mindful eating habits, balanced macronutrient intake, and a focus on nutrient-dense foods. By incorporating a variety of eating habits like plant-based, low-carb, intermittent fasting, and more, we can support our bodies and minds as we age. It is important to listen to our bodies, pay attention to our hunger cues, and make choices that support our health and wellness in the long term.

Macro-Friendly Meal Planning

Macro-Friendly Meal Planning is a key aspect of maintaining a healthy and fit lifestyle in your 40's. By focusing on the balance of macronutrients - protein, carbohydrates, and fats - you can ensure that your body is getting the fuel it needs to thrive. This approach can help you achieve and maintain a healthy weight, support muscle maintenance, and provide sustained energy throughout the day.

When planning your meals, be sure to include a good source of lean protein, such as chicken, fish, tofu, or legumes. Protein is essential for muscle maintenance and repair, as well as keeping you feeling full and satisfied. Aim to include protein in each meal and snack to support your overall health and fitness goals.

In addition to protein, be mindful of your carbohydrate intake. While carbohydrates are an important source of energy, it's important to choose complex carbohydrates such as whole grains, fruits, and vegetables over refined sugars and processed foods. By focusing on high-quality carbohydrates, you can support stable blood sugar levels and avoid energy crashes throughout the day.

When it comes to fats, opt for healthy sources such as avocados, nuts, seeds, and olive oil. These fats are essential for brain health, hormone production, and nutrient absorption. Including a variety of healthy fats in your diet can support overall wellness and help you feel your best in your 40's.

By following a macro-friendly meal plan, you can ensure that your body is getting the nutrients it needs to thrive. Whether you're focused on weight management, muscle maintenance, or overall wellness, balancing your macronutrients is key. With a focus on lean protein, complex carbohydrates, and healthy fats, you can support your health and fitness goals in your 40's and beyond.

Chapter 11: Superfood-Focused Eating Habits for Boosting Immunity in Your 40's

What Are Superfoods?

Superfoods are a category of nutrient-dense foods that are particularly beneficial for our health and well-being. These foods are packed with vitamins, minerals, antioxidants, and other essential nutrients that can help boost our immunity, support our weight management goals, and improve our overall health. Including superfoods in your diet can be a great way to ensure that you are getting the nutrients your body needs to thrive, especially as you enter your 40s.

One of the key benefits of superfoods is their ability to boost our immune system. As we age, our immune system may weaken, making us more susceptible to illnesses and infections. Superfoods like berries, leafy greens, and nuts are rich in antioxidants and phytonutrients that can help strengthen our immune defences and protect us from harmful pathogens. By incorporating these superfoods into your diet, you can give your immune system the support it needs to keep you healthy and strong.

Another important aspect of superfoods is their role in weight management. Many superfoods are low in calories but high in nutrients, making them an excellent choice for those looking to maintain a healthy weight. Superfoods like quinoa, chia seeds, and avocados are rich in fibre and protein, which can help keep you feeling full and satisfied, while also providing you with essential nutrients for optimal health. By including these superfoods in your diet, you can support your weight management goals and feel your best in your 40s.

Superfoods are also known for their anti-inflammatory properties, which can help reduce the risk of chronic diseases and improve overall health. Inflammation is a natural response in the body, but chronic inflammation can lead to a variety of health issues, including heart disease, diabetes, and arthritis. Superfoods like turmeric, ginger, and fatty fish are rich in anti-inflammatory compounds that can help reduce inflammation in the body and promote better health. By incorporating these superfoods into your diet, you can help reduce inflammation and support your body in staying healthy and strong as you age.

In conclusion, superfoods are a valuable addition to any diet, especially for those in their 40s who are looking to maintain their health and well-being. By incorporating a variety of superfoods into your meals, you can boost your immunity, support your weight management goals, reduce inflammation, and improve your overall health. Whether you choose to include berries, leafy greens, nuts, or fatty fish, adding superfoods to your diet can help you feel your best and stay healthy and fit in your 40s and beyond.

Immune-Boosting Superfoods to Add to Your Diet

Incorporating immune-boosting superfoods into your diet is essential for maintaining a strong and healthy body, especially as you age into your 40s. These nutrient-dense foods are packed with vitamins, minerals, antioxidants, and other compounds that support your immune system and help ward off illness. By adding these superfoods to your daily meals, you can give your body the extra boost it needs to stay healthy and fit.

One superfood that is particularly beneficial for boosting immunity is garlic. Garlic contains allicin, a compound that has been shown to have antimicrobial properties and can help fight off infections. Adding garlic to your meals or taking a garlic supplement can help support your immune system and keep you feeling your best. Other superfoods that are great for immunity include ginger, turmeric, and green tea, all of which have powerful anti-inflammatory and antioxidant properties.

Berries are another group of superfoods that can help boost your immune system. Berries like blueberries, strawberries, and raspberries are rich in vitamin C, which is known for its immune-boosting properties. These fruits also contain flavonoids, which have been shown to help reduce inflammation and support overall immune function. Adding a variety of berries to your diet can help keep your immune system strong and resilient.

Leafy green vegetables, such as spinach, kale, and Swiss chard, are also excellent immune-boosting superfoods. These greens are rich in vitamins A, C, and E, as well as antioxidants like beta-carotene and lutein. These nutrients help support your immune system by reducing inflammation and promoting the production of white blood cells, which are essential for fighting off infections. Incorporating leafy greens into your meals can help keep your immune system strong and your body healthy.

In addition to these superfoods, it's important to maintain a balanced and varied diet that includes a wide range of nutrients to support overall wellness. By incorporating immune-boosting superfoods like garlic, berries, and leafy greens into your meals, you can give your body the extra support it needs to stay healthy and strong in your 40s and beyond. Remember to also prioritize other healthy eating habits, such as staying hydrated, getting enough sleep, and managing stress, to keep your immune system functioning at its best.

Superfood Recipes for Immunity

Superfoods are nutrient-dense foods that are packed with vitamins, minerals, and antioxidants that can help boost your immune system and keep you healthy and fit in your 40's. Incorporating superfoods into your diet is a great way to support your body's natural defences and promote overall wellness. In this subchapter, we will explore some delicious superfood recipes that can help you strengthen your immunity and stay healthy as you age.

One superfood recipe that is perfect for boosting immunity is a green smoothie packed with spinach, kale, avocado, and berries. These ingredients are rich in vitamins C and E, as well as antioxidants that can help protect your cells from damage and strengthen your immune system. Simply blend all the ingredients together with some almond milk or coconut water for a delicious and nutritious beverage that will keep you feeling energized and healthy.

Another superfood recipe that can help support your immune system is a quinoa salad with roasted vegetables and chickpeas. Quinoa is a complete protein that is rich in fibre and essential amino acids, while the roasted vegetables and chickpeas provide a variety of vitamins and minerals that can help keep your immune system strong. Toss the cooked quinoa with the roasted vegetables and chickpeas, along with some olive oil, lemon juice, and fresh herbs for a satisfying and nutritious meal that will keep you feeling full and satisfied.

Turmeric is another powerful superfood that can help boost your immunity and reduce inflammation in your body. One delicious way to incorporate turmeric into your diet is by making a golden milk latte with almond milk, turmeric, ginger, and cinnamon. Turmeric contains a compound called curcumin, which has been shown to have anti-inflammatory and antioxidant properties that can help support your immune system and promote overall wellness. Simply heat up the almond milk with the turmeric, ginger, and cinnamon, and enjoy a soothing and immune-boosting beverage that is perfect for relaxing in the evening.

Incorporating superfoods into your diet is a simple and effective way to support your immune system and stay healthy and fit in your 40's. By including nutrient-dense foods like spinach, kale, berries, quinoa, turmeric, and more into your meals, you can help strengthen your body's natural defences and promote overall wellness. Try out these superfood recipes and see how they can help boost your immunity and keep you feeling healthy and strong as you age.

Chapter 12: Conclusion - Making Healthy Eating Habits a Lifestyle Choice at 40

In conclusion, making healthy eating habits a lifestyle choice at 40 is essential for maintaining a strong body and mind. As we age, our bodies require more nutrients to support optimal health and prevent the onset of chronic diseases. By adopting a plant-based eating habit, you can ensure that you are getting a variety of vitamins, minerals, and antioxidants that are essential for overall wellness. Plant-based diets have been shown to reduce the risk of heart disease, diabetes, and certain types of cancer, making them an ideal choice for those in their 40s looking to prioritize their health.

Another beneficial eating habit for those in their 40s is following a low-carb diet for weight management. By reducing your intake of carbohydrates and focusing on protein and healthy fats, you can promote weight loss and improve your body composition. Low-carb diets have also been linked to lower blood sugar levels and improved insulin sensitivity, making them a great choice for those looking to prevent or manage diabetes. Additionally, intermittent fasting can be a useful tool for increasing energy levels and promoting weight loss in your 40s.

For those concerned about heart health, adopting a Mediterranean diet can be highly beneficial. This eating habit focuses on consuming plenty of fruits, vegetables, whole grains, and healthy fats like olive oil and nuts. The Mediterranean diet has been shown to reduce the risk of heart disease, stroke, and cognitive decline, making it an excellent choice for those in their 40s looking to support their cardiovascular health. Additionally, incorporating gluten-free eating habits can help improve digestive health and reduce inflammation in the body.

In order to maintain muscle mass and strength in your 40s, it is important to focus on protein-rich eating habits. Protein is essential for building and repairing muscle tissue, as well as supporting a healthy immune system. By including sources of lean protein like chicken, fish, tofu, and legumes in your diet, you can ensure that your body has the nutrients it needs to stay strong and healthy. Additionally, reducing your intake of sugar can help reduce inflammation in the body and support overall wellness in your 40s.

Mindful eating habits can also be beneficial for managing stress and promoting mental well-being in your 40s. By paying attention to your hunger cues, eating slowly, and savouring each bite, you can improve digestion, reduce overeating, and enhance your overall relationship with food. Finally, focusing on a balanced macro-nutrient eating habit can help ensure that you are getting all the nutrients your body needs for optimal health. By including a variety of carbohydrates, proteins, and fats in your diet, you can support your energy levels, muscle maintenance, and overall wellness in your 40s. Additionally, incorporating superfood-focused eating habits can help boost your immunity and protect against illness and disease. By making healthy eating habits a priority in your 40s, you can set yourself up for a vibrant and fulfilling life.

www.ingramcontent.com/pod-product-compliance
Lightning Source LLC
Chambersburg PA
CBHW051706250726
48653CB00007B/2883